Glycemic Index Diet

A Proven Diet Plan For Weight Loss and Healthy Eating With No Calorie Counting

By Susan T. Williams

This book is designed to provide information on the topic covered. The information herein is offered for informational purposes solely. It is sold with the understanding that neither the author nor the publisher is engaged in rendering legal, accounting or other professional services. If legal or other professional advice is warranted, the services of an appropriate professional should be sought.

While every effort has been made to make the information presented here as complete and accurate as possible, it may contain errors, omissions or information that was accurate as of its publication but subsequently has become outdated by marketplace or industry changes. Neither author nor publisher accepts any liability or responsibility to any person or entity with respect to any loss or damage alleged to have been caused, directly or indirectly, by the information, ideas, opinions or other content in this book.

In no way, is it legal to reproduce, duplicate, or transmit any part of this document in either electronic means or printed form. Recording of this publication is strictly prohibited and any storage of this document is not allowed unless with written permission from the publisher.
The use of any trademark within this book is for clarifying purposes only, and any trademarks referenced in this work are used are without consent, and remain the property of the respective trademark holders, who are not affiliated with the publisher or this book.

Table of Contents

Introduction

A re you familiar with the glycemic index but want to learn more or is it an entirely new concept to you? Either way, we are about to show you how the glycemic index is calculated and how natural foods can stabilize your blood sugar levels and give you added health benefits too – one of them being radical weight loss.

You get to understand how controlling the foods you eat based on the glycemic index can result in weight loss, reduce the risk of diabetes and lower your cholesterol.

The glycemic diet is not just another fad diet.

When you use the glycemic index to plan your meals, it means that you are actually following a glycemic index diet. What may come as a surprise to you is that the GI diet is not a "diet" where you have to follow specific meal plans, lists of foods to eat and foods to avoid; rather, it's a way of life. The glycemic index is a tool and proven method you can use to select foods that meet your specific dietary needs and desires.

The glycemic index measures carbohydrates, which are made up of simple or complex sugar molecules. It also ranks food depending on the rate at which the body breaks it down to form glucose.

The goal of this ebook is to help you understand these effects and adhere to the simple guidelines that will help you recognize foods by their glycemic index. The ebook will also help you to make better food choices.

Carbohydrates have earned a bad rap, but they are not really the villains they are made out to be. Many carbohydrates are good for you, and it is not necessary to avoid all carbohydrates, as many fad diets suggest.

As you read on, you see how high and low blood sugar levels can affect your health and your feelings of well being. You are able to identify the direct link between GI and controlling diabetes. You may even be able to substantially reduce the risk of becoming diabetic.

This book also includes a list of many common foods and their GI rating together with easy-to-follow suggestions that will allow you to make the right food choices. You can then use the glycemic index to make gradual, lasting changes in your diet, at which point, you will realize that making the best food choices comes naturally to you.

We won't pretend that it's an easy journey. It will take a lot of work on your part to learn good dietary practices and change how you think about food. The end result is certainly well worth the effort.

CHAPTER 1

The Glycemic Index—An Overview

The GI concept was originally developed in 1981 by Canadian professor and scientist, Dr. David Jenkins, along with his colleagues at the University of Toronto. It was designed mainly to help people with diabetes. GI is now also promoted for weight loss and overall wellbeing. The idea behind GI is to make sure people consume foods that are digested more slowly in order to promote greater satiety. Being satisfied after a meal also helps people to eat less.

Glycemic Index—How does it work?

GI, which stands for glycemic index, is a number. This number is assigned to a given food, mainly carbohydrates, based on how fast its sugars and starches are digested and absorbed into the bloodstream when compared with pure glucose. So, this means that a low GI indicates that the food is digested and absorbed more slowly.

Seeing the popularity of diets like South Beach and Atkins, which vilified all carbohydrates and fats, Dr. Jenkins felt the need to develop a better system. He could not accept the oversimplified way in which carbohydrates were categorized as "good carbohydrates" and "bad carbohydrates or "simple" versus "complex". His research proves that carbohydrates are complex and that all foods affect your bodies' blood sugar levels differently.

Food breaks down in your digestive system into several components such as sugar, minerals and vitamins. These different components ultimately get absorbed into your blood stream. They have an immediate impact on your system. Some foods which break down rapidly and have high glucose or sugar levels give you a "sugar high", something that feels like a rush of energy. These are high GI foods, and they break down quickly. You feel hungry soon and are left looking for the next food fix.

Foods that break down at a slower pace, releasing their sugars and nutrients over a longer period of time, do not cause any sudden spike to your sugar levels. Your insulin levels remain low and steady. Low GI foods break down more slowly. You can eat less without feeling hungry for a longer period of time when you eat low GI foods. You feel satisfied with less. These low GI foods form the core of the glycemic index diet.

As you read on, you will find out exactly what glucose and insulin are and how they affect your body and health. Through his research, Dr. Jenkins proved that many carbohydrates were, in fact, very good for you and should not be avoided just because they are carbohydrates.

He found that several foods that were categorized as unhealthy in the past were actually very beneficial. On the other hand, some foods that had always been considered "diet" foods displayed a high GI.

Dr. Jenkins continues his study in the field of dietary science and carries on his pursuit of learning more about the connection between diet and health. He believes that following certain dietary patterns can improve or eliminate the risk of health issues such as diabetes, cancer and heart disease.

GI can be high or low.

Most foods that are ranked higher on the GI index, such as those made from white flour, are heavily processed. These foods have been stripped of all their essential nutrients. On the other hand, low GI foods like vegetables, fruits, nuts, whole grains, legumes, low-fat dairy and lean meat and fish, are real, wholesome foods rich in nutrients that are essential for good health.

The GI diet does the math for you.

Following the GI diet is pretty easy. All foods can be classified in three color categories that follow the traffic signal colors: food listed under red should be avoided if you want to lose weight; yellow light foods can be enjoyed occasionally; and green light foods can be eaten to your heart's content.

The GI Diet will never leave you feeling starved or deprived. It is as easy as the traffic signal system—if you can follow traffic signals, you will find the GI Diet easy to follow. Unlike some of the impractical to downright dangerous diets, the GI diet will not in affect your health adversely. Instead, it will reduce your risk of type 2 diabetes, heart disease, stroke and cancer.

CHAPTER 2

Measuring the Glycemic Index of foods

Pure glucose or white bread is the control food or standard that the glycemic index uses to measure and rate other carbohydrates. The standard is given a GI of "100", and all other foods are tested to find how they affect your blood sugar levels in comparison to it. The GI value of a food is measured by feeding 10 or more healthy people (the test subjects) a food containing 50 grams of glucose or white bread and then measuring the effect on their blood glucose levels over the next two hours.

The next step is to take the same test subjects and ask them to eat a sample of the food that needs to be tested. Their two-hour blood glucose response is then calculated. The results are measured after all the tests have been completed. The results are graphed and measured to find out how the food affects the person's blood sugar levels in relation to the glucose.

A number rating is given to each tested food and it is classified as either "High", "Medium" or "Low" on the glycemic index. Foods rated as having a High GI would have a rating of 70 or above. Low GI food items will be rated at 55 or lower. All food that falls within the 56 to 69 range would be rated as Medium GI foods.

The GI values of foods must be determined using valid scientific methods, and one cannot guess the GI value of a food just by looking at the composition of the food. Currently, there are only a few nutrition research groups around the world that are authorized to provide a valid GI testing service.

The amount of food that the test subject has to consume would depend on the food that is being tested. Foods that are dense in carbohydrates would require a small sample size; whereas an enormous amount of food would need to be eaten by the test subject if the sample had very little carbohydrates in it.

What affects a food item's Glycemic Index?

Many factors determine the GI of a food.

- *How you cook*

The type of heat, amount of water and cooking time can alter a food's GI. The starch granules are expanded to varying degrees by the water and heat during the cooking process. Boiled or baked potatoes have higher GI's and are easily digested when compared to whole wheat pasta, even though both are starchy foods.

This is because during the process of boiling or baking the potatoes, the starch gets gelatinized (or swollen) to the bursting point, thus making it easily digestible. This is not the case with the less gelatinized starch in whole wheat pasta. The GI of a baked potato is 85 and whole wheat pasta is 32.

• *Type of starch*

Starches consist of two molecules that connect together to form starch granules. These are called amylose and amylopectin, and each of them displays different characteristics that have different effects on GI. Molecules of amylose are harder to digest than molecules of amylopectin. Foods which are low on amylose and high on amylopectin have higher GI values. For example, wheat flour and jasmine rice have more amylopectin starch molecules which are easily gelatinized during cooking and are digested easily by the body.

Foods with more amylose have lower GI values, such as legumes and basmati rice, and are therefore harder to digest.

• *How it is processed*

Processing starchy food by grinding, milling or rolling reduces the particle size, making it easier for water and digestive enzymes to penetrate. Grains also lose their fibrous outer coat when they are processed, and this allows enzymes easy access to the starch. Flours that are finely milled have smaller particles and therefore a higher GI than coarsely ground flours.

• *Type of sugar present*

Sugar, or sucrose, is made up of glucose and fructose. Fructose has a lower GI (68) than glucose, which has a GI of 100. Digestion of sugar produces only half the amount of glucose molecules, with the other half being fructose, which is known to attract a very small blood sugar response. Sugar also inhibits the gelatinization of starch by binding with the water molecules, thereby reducing the amount of water that is available. Breakfast cereals and oatmeal cookies are some examples of this.

• *Type of fiber present*

Fibers that are viscous and soluble increase the viscosity of the contents in the digestive tract. This results in slowing down the action of the enzymes on the starch. A lower blood sugar response is created, and therefore these foods have a lower GI.

Lentils and rolled oats contain soluble fiber and have low GIs. However, since finely milled wheat flour does not have viscous fiber, it gets digested quickly and has a high GI.

• *Fat content*

Fat slows the rate at which the food leaves the stomach. Foods containing fat may cause a rise in blood sugar by slowing the digestion of carbohydrates in the intestine. This is why foods containing fat, such as potato chips, have a lower GI of 57 while similar foods without fat, like baked potato, have a GI of 85.

But wait! This certainly does not make it okay to reach for that bag of potato chips in your bottom drawer. While baked potato is very low in saturated fat, it is an excellent source of vitamin C, potassium, vitamin B6 and manganese, whereas potato chips are heavily processed and lack nutrition of any kind.

- *Acidity of the food*

The presence of acids in food results in a slowdown of the rate at which your stomach empties. This further increases the time it takes to digest carbohydrates. Adding acids to your meal does result in a lower GI and changes the blood sugar response. Some examples of this are adding vinegar or lemon juice to foods in the form of pickles or salad dressings and eating sourdough bread.

CHAPTER 3

Why all carbs are not created equal

Very often carbohydrates take the blame for weight gain, diabetes, and just about anything else that is wrong in one's diet. Popular opinion usually blames carbohydrates for the rising rate of obesity, and studies have shown that low carb diets do result in long term weight loss and a reduction in the occurrence of diabetes.

Most people discuss carbohydrates without really understanding what they are or knowing their significance in the diet. Over the years, dieticians and doctors have attacked the base of the food pyramid. The bottom level of the food pyramid consists of different forms of carbohydrates— bread, cereal, rice and pasta. They claim that these foods are the cause of the increasing obesity we see in the US and many other parts of the world. Ever since a doctor named Atkins claimed that carbohydrates are evil, several variations of the low carb diet have been recycled. It is easy for anyone to fall for the common belief that carbs are indeed the enemy.

Get over the carb phobia.

Carbohydrates are not all the same. They come in a variety of forms. Some are good for you and some are not. The ones that are not good for you are usually highly processed. These food items can barely be described as food. They may be yummy, but they're also the result of some crazy chemical processes.

The food industry has been quick to catch on to carb mania. We now have an array of low carb packaged food as well as restaurant menus with low carb items, both of which are fashionable and popular.

Jenkins proves that different carbohydrates affect your blood sugar levels and release insulin to different degrees. Carbohydrates can have a high glycemic index or a low one. Many carbohydrates which are thought of as "bad" really weren't, and some others that were considered "healthy" would cause a sharp rise in blood sugar levels.

Watermelon has a very high GI of 72, but is also an extremely good source of vitamin C, magnesium, vitamin B1 and vitamin B6. It has a high GI because its high sugar content raises your blood sugar levels and forces your body to release insulin to counteract and lower these levels. Insulin lowers your blood sugar and leaves you feeling irritable and lethargic. That's when you find yourself outside your neighborhood donut shop, falling in line to pick up a dozen chocolate donuts. Your falling blood sugar levels make you hungrier faster.

CHAPTER 4

The facts about sugar

Your body's energy is mostly produced from carbohydrates. Molecules of sugar are broken down and converted into oxygen and carbon dioxide molecules. These molecules are the energy or fuel that keeps your body functioning. This conversion translates into your metabolism. How fast or slow your metabolism is depends on how efficiently your body can turn food into energy.

When you consume food which contains easily obtainable carbohydrates, your blood sugar levels rise, and this may increase your risk of diabetes, obesity and heart disease. Sudden increase in blood sugar can also make you sleepy once your levels come back to normal.

It's all about keeping your blood sugar levels balanced.

Glucose, a simple sugar found in many foods, is one of the primary sources of energy. It allows your organs and your brain to function properly. Remember that buzz you get after drinking a soda?

Many feel dizzy and lightheaded when their blood sugar levels go too high or too low. Your body tries to maintain a balance, and when you overfeed it with sugar or deprive it of carbohydrates, it will try to overcompensate. Your body will then release insulin to try to compensate for what you've eaten.

And that's when you will feel symptoms. Initially, you will feel the immediate reaction from either too much glucose consumed or the effects of under eating. After this, you will experience the counteractions that your body has to perform.

Several things can help keep your blood sugar levels balanced. Regularly spaced meals and snacks and daily exercise help, but your food choices are the key.

Selecting your meals or snacks based on their GI helps you to find foods that will keep your blood sugar low. The lower the GI ranking of the food item, the less of an impact on your blood sugar levels. Foods with a low GI ranking have a milder effect on blood sugar level because they are digested by your body slowly.

So, when you eat foods that have a GI below 55, blood sugar levels are raised only slightly. Consuming foods which have a GI between t 55-70 will raise your blood sugar levels a little higher. Eating foods with a GI above 70 will cause a sudden spike in your blood sugar levels.

Studies prove that a low GI Diet can be more satisfying than a high GI one. Low GI meals help to control overeating, which can lead to weight loss. Experts also assert that a low GI Diet can prevent the development of insulin resistance. Insulin resistance is one of the key factors in developing diabetes.

Since insulin resistance can lead to weight gain around the waist, a known risk factor for cardiovascular disease, a low GI diet may also protect you from heart disease.

Insulin is the key.

Your pancreas produces a hormone called insulin. Insulin acts like the waistband of your trousers— it lets your body's cells know when they have been fed sufficiently and have received an ample supply of nutrients.

Insulin mainly works to control the metabolism of carbohydrates, lipids and proteins. It also moderates the function and growth of the body's cells. Once you have eaten a meal, insulin routes the excess glucose and stores it in your liver in the form of glycogen. The liver releases glycogen into your bloodstream in the form of sugar when the insulin levels are low, especially between meals.

So, when you consume too many sugars, proteins or fats, your body hoards the excess in order to burn it when your body needs energy. It does not use the extra fat deposits you already store in your body.

Constantly eating food high on the glycemic index will force your body to release insulin continuously. Overworking your insulin and making it react to large amounts of glucose leads to a condition called "insulin resistance." When this happens, your insulin production just can't keep up with the massive workload, and the body's cells become resistant to the effects of insulin.

Over time, insulin resistance can cause type 2 diabetes because the beta cells are not able to keep up with your body's increased requirement for insulin. Your body cannot digest and reroute the excess glucose or any other kind of sugars or carbs that build up in the bloodstream. You then have to provide your body with an artificial regulator. You would need to get insulin injections every day.

Diabetes presents your body with enormous complications. We will discuss diabetes in details in the following chapters. If you are not well informed about diabetes, it is very important that you take time to read up on the subject. Educating yourself about this condition is the right way to ensure that you live a healthy life.

But you have not been diagnosed with diabetes, you say.

You also have no family history of diabetes. However, you will still benefit from understanding what you can do to reduce your risk of developing diabetes. Genetic factors aside, diabetes is also known as a lifestyle disease, that is to say, it is a disease caused by civilization. This disease can lead to many serious complications and even untimely death.

But there is no need to worry. You can use the GI as a guide in selecting foods for meal planning and coming up with a diabetes diet by which you may avoid the risk of developing diabetes altogether. Let's proceed on to learn more about how you can avoid diabetes with a glycemic index diet.

CHAPTER 5

The GI and the reduced risk of Diabetes

By now, you understand that sugar can raise your blood sugar levels to dangerous highs. And sugar lurks in more places than just sweet treats like ice cream and pecan pies. Your seemingly healthy dinner plates, laden with pasta and potatoes, are loaded with sugar too.

All foods containing carbohydrates will have sugars, fibers and starches, even though they may not be sweet. Your favorite foods that aren't sweet to your taste buds may actually contain loads of glucose. French fries or the delicious garlic shrimp noodles you ordered from the Chinese restaurant next door can raise your blood sugar levels very high. This makes your body's insulin levels shoot up as well.

Consuming too much sugar makes heavy demands on your insulin producing cells. It wears them out. Over time, insulin stops responding to the high blood sugar levels and finally, insulin production eventually stops.

Could it be diabetes?

Diabetes is of two types, type 1 and type 2. The onset of diabetes symptoms is due to a higher level of glucose in your blood. Very often, the signs are mild. You may not notice these signs, particularly in type 2 diabetes. You may not realize what is happening until it's too late. The symptoms caused by type 1 diabetes are more severe.

Diabetes warning signs:

Hunger and tiredness: Since your insulin is ineffective, your body continuously breaks down the food that you eat into sugars. However, these sugars are not converted to energy.

Thirst and frequent urination: It's not unusual to urinate four to seven times in a day, but people with diabetes may need to go a lot more. This is because your body pushes out all the extra glucose through your urine. It needs to make more urine to get rid of the sugar that your body is not able to absorb. So, you urinate more frequently. And when you urinate so frequently, you feel thirsty and your fluid intake increases.

Dry mouth and itchiness: Your body uses all the fluids you drink to flush out the excess glucose in the form of urine. This causes dehydration in your body, which is why your mouth and skin can become dry. In the case of dry skin, you may experience itchiness as well.

Blurry vision: This is caused by the change in the fluid levels in your body. The lens in your eyes swells up and changes shape. This makes them lose the ability to focus.

More about diabetes

Type 1 diabetes is the more complicated of the two. It is critical that you manage it properly in order to prevent short or long term complications. If you have developed type 1 diabetes, the beta cells in your pancreas are damaged. They are no longer able to make the insulin required to counteract your blood sugar levels.

The main sources of energy for your body are sugar and starch, and they are present in most foods. Since it is not possible to avoid foods that raise your blood sugar, your body will not be able to survive for long without insulin. It starts to malfunction, as it is not able to handle the incoming energy.

Artificial insulin needs to be supplied on a regular basis through injections, so that your body can process glucose. It is important to have constant awareness of what you are eating. You also must monitor your blood sugar levels several times a day.

Type 2 diabetes is more common, and is different from Type 1 diabetes because the body is able to produce insulin. However, the quantity produced is not enough. In some cases, the insulin that is produced is not effective. Many type 2 diabetics are able to manage their condition by following a strict diabetic diet, exercising and utilizing oral medication.

Type 2 diabetes is a progressive condition. If you do not control it carefully, your condition may deteriorate with time. You may even need to inject insulin, which will help your body process sugar and prevent long term complications. Your condition can be exacerbated if you consume high GI foods, and it could even cause failure of the insulin response.

It's never too late to start a GI diet.

You do not have to stay away from carbohydrates and foods containing sugar if you are not a diabetic. But it is important that you remember to moderate your consumption. The best bet is to consume plenty of low GI foods. You can eat less of the medium GI foods and occasionally treat yourself to high GI foods.

If you are a diabetic, you already know that any food that has carbohydrates can raise your blood sugar—that goes for organic brown rice as well as cheese fries. You can take some simple steps while planning your meals to help keep your blood sugar in check.

How do low GI foods affect diabetes?

Low GI foods tend to break down more slowly. When you consume low GI foods, it is less likely that there will be a rapid increase in your blood sugar levels. Low GI foods are a better option for maintaining stable blood glucose levels.

Opting for a GI diet that is rich in low GI foods rather than high GI foods leaves you feeling more satisfied over a longer period of time. You are less likely to feel hungry before your next meal.

How do high GI foods affect diabetes?

Foods that are high GI break down rapidly. This causes a sharp rise in your blood glucose levels. High GI foods will also force the body to work overtime and produce larger quantities of insulin to process the quick acting carbohydrates.

The result? You start getting hunger pangs within 2 to 3 hours. This is particularly dangerous for diabetics because your body's ability to control blood glucose is greatly reduced. Diabetics need to be extremely careful when they consume high GI foods.

Lower the GI of your diabetes diet easily.

Favor more fiber: Bring out the black bean stew and the oatmeal casserole. Dish up the bulgur and lentil pilaf. Most often, the more fiber in a food, the lower the GI. Fiber adds bulk to your diet. It aids good digestion as well as elimination. High fiber foods are slow to digest, and so they help to stabilize your blood sugar. Make sure to include both soluble and insoluble fiber. The soluble fiber is the kind you find in fruits, vegetables and oats which help you feel full after your meal. Insoluble fiber behaves like a "sweep" that aids in moving food through your colon easily and helps you maintain healthy and regular bowel movements.

Keep away from processed food: When food is processed, it gets digested faster. These foods have high GIs. Corn flakes pack a bigger punch than an ear of sweet corn, and instant oatmeal will spike your blood sugar more than steel cut oats. The simple rule to remember is that the closer a food is to its natural state; the better it is for you.

Combine and consume: Reduce the impact of food that has a high GI by combining it with some low GI food. If you're having baked potato, which has a high GI, combine it with a salad, which has a low GI. This lowers the overall GI to an average value.

Similarly, if you plan to have moderate glycemic food such as beans for lunch, add a side of a low glycemic food like an avocado or turkey. Eating beans with a high glycemic food such as rice would only raise the glycemic response. This would be disastrous for blood sugar control.

Scrimp on potatoes: Potatoes are packed with carbohydrates that quickly convert to sugar and enter the blood stream. Enjoy small portions but not too often. Avoid mashed potatoes. Mashing increases the GI by 25 percent because it is easier to break down when compared to boiled potatoes.

A dash of vinegar: Perk up your meal with a little vinegar or lemon juice. Acids lower a meal's GI.

Quality and quantity: The quantity or portion size matters when it comes to managing your blood glucose. The GI value only represents the type of carbohydrate in the food.

Nutrition matters: Many high GI foods are nutritious, while low GI foods are not. Example, instant oatmeal has a GI of 83 whereas dark chocolate has a GI of 23. This does not mean you can have a whole slab of dark chocolate for breakfast. The principles of GI need to be balanced with that of basic nutrition.

Studying and understanding a basic glycemic index (GI) chart can be very helpful in forming a basic diet plan. (See a list of over 150 foods and their glycemic index ranking.) Focus on food types which are lowest on the glycemic chart, which are rich in proteins and healthy fats. Enjoy some fibrous vegetables, nuts and seeds. Combine moderate GI foods such as beans and legumes together with low glycemic foods.

Evaluate fruits carefully. Consume fruits that are low on the glycemic chart like apples, berries and citrus fruits. Of course, it is important to assess the amount of carbohydrates and protein you are consuming in the context of your total caloric intake. Using the GI as a framework can help make life easier and prevent stringent calorie counting.

Aim to obtain at least 80% of your calories from low GI (under 30) foods. Fill the remaining 20% of your plate with moderate glycemic foods, in proper combination. Remember always that high GI foods are essentially toxic to those suffering from diabetes.

You can almost eliminate the risk of contracting diabetes by following the GI diet. By protecting your insulin response from being over worked, the GI Diet keeps your heart, brain and other organs healthier, even if you have a history of diabetes in your family.

Eating low GI foods will allow your internal systems and organs to work at their optimal capacity, and you will look as good as you feel on the inside. Add 30 minutes of moderate exercise every day, and you can help stave off diabetes altogether.

CHAPTER 6

The GI path to Weight Loss

Sure, eating the right types of food will help you to avoid heart disease and protect your gallbladder. But what wouldn't you do to drop a pant size or a dress size or two? While the main reason for developing the GI was to guide diabetics to make appropriate food choices, a low-glycemic diet has been connected to weight loss as well.

Most diet plans are all about counting calories. They lay down rules that you need to live your life by. Some diet plans are so stringent; they could be called diet boot camps. The GI diet goes beyond calories; it is a way of life.

It urges you to see how foods are prepared, digested and metabolized in your body. It makes you pay attention to what impact everything you eat has on your weight. It makes you observe how full you feel after eating. There's no one right way to follow a GI diet to lose weight. Nor is there a black-and-white approach where you're "on" or "off" the diet.

So you say that science was never one of your strong points in school. But that's okay, because the GI is based on several detailed scientific studies that categorize foods based on their effect on blood sugar and insulin. The GI itself is not a diet plan but one of the various tools to guide you in making the best food choices that help you in your objective to lose weight. You use the information in the GI list to add additional healthy benefits to your food choices.

Glycemic diet—a simple, doable weight-loss tool.

The GI Diet teaches you to make food choices that allow you to lose weight naturally – and even better, keep it off easily. This is because by following a low GI diet, you choose foods that keep your sugar and insulin levels on a healthy and constant plateau. These are the same food types that give you a longer, more constant feeling of fullness and satiation. Your energy levels are kept "fed" continuously. You don't feel the need to keep eating.

Remember that incredible feeling of euphoria after tucking into a hot, crisp glazed donut? You should also recall the low that followed it, which at that time, you may have attributed to the unread emails in your inbox at work. This "bottoming out" is for real. It happens each time you gorge on a sugary delight. You may put your body through this sort of situation so often that you don't even recognize it.

You wonder why you are hungry again within minutes of eating something that was made up of food belonging to the high end of the glycemic index. High GI foods take your body on a roller coaster ride. These steep ups and downs will destroy your health and keep you from losing weight successfully.

If you maintain a low GI diet, your insulin may become more responsive and sensitive. When your insulin is able to react rapidly and efficiently to anything you eat, you will find yourself losing weight, start getting into better shape and become healthier than before. A low GI diet acts as a workout for your insulin.

A low GI diet helps you to lose weight by controlling your appetite and by promoting satiety. High GI food causes a rapid increase in blood glucose, which is followed by a rapid insulin response and a subsequent return to feeling hungry. Low GI foods work by delaying feelings of hunger. And it's not hard to believe that you lose weight when you eat less, right?

How can you lose weight with a low GI Diet?

Initially, you may not find it easy to follow a low GI Diet rigidly. For one thing, it's difficult to know what to eat unless you carry an extensive list around with you. You could certainly use a glycemic index list as a weight-loss tool by selecting low-glycemic foods. You can even balance out a high glycemic food choice with a lower GI one.

Here's how you can lose weight by following a low GI diet.

- Substitute as many high GI foods with healthy lower GI alternatives as possible. For example, substitute instant oatmeal with old-fashioned oats, which have a higher percentage of fiber as well as hard, compact starch granules when compared to instant oatmeal. Most of the starches in the instant oatmeal are processed and therefore are easily digested.
- Include at least one healthy low GI food at each meal. If you are having a sandwich for lunch, make sure it has a low GI filling, like turkey or chicken with a spread like hummus or tomato and cilantro chutney.
- Keep away from refined flours. They are not good for you. Always choose low GI whole grains.
- Combine high GI foods with low GI foods to reduce the blood sugar impact. For example, bring life to your bagels by topping it with thinly sliced cucumber and tomato. Drizzle balsamic vinegar for a zing and sprinkle some ground black pepper for extra flavor.
- Always control portions. No matter what they contain, big meals always trigger a higher blood glucose response than smaller ones. Never super-size your meals.

Using a GI diet to lose weight will definitely take some time and some hard work at first. But once you learn to focus on how eating high GI foods make you feel, following the glycemic index will be effortless.

CHAPTER 7

The GI path to improving Heart Health

By now, you understand that the GI is a helpful tool for diabetics, in particular, because it helps to assess the blood sugar-raising effects of various foods. Foods with lower GI have a lesser impact on your blood sugar. And this is the ultimate goal for people suffering from diabetes.

Diabetics often tend to have cardiovascular complications that usually involve problems with cholesterol and high blood pressure.

Heart diseases and GI—Is there a connection?

You may find it hard to imagine a connection between eating foods high in starches and sugars and heart disease. The connection is most definitely there. Each time you feast on foods that have a high GI, your entire system has to go on a hyperactive mode in order to bring it back down to more normal functioning.

It's simple. Your body's main sources of energy are sugars and starches. When you eat food containing sugars, your body will try to use it or store it if it is not needed at that moment. Overindulging in high GI foods taxes your body to work harder, and every system in the body starts to feel the burden. Your blood pressure rises so that the sugar and insulin can be moved in the bloodstream as fast as possible. Your heart becomes super active in order to keep the blood flowing and to increase the oxygen needed to perform all needed functions.

Even people who run marathons and cycle long distances are at a risk of suffering long-term damage to their hearts. Therefore, it isn't hard to imagine when the heart of a person who continuously feeds their body with unhealthy food fails.

Save your heart. Consume more low GI foods.

If you have high cholesterol, eating a low GI diet is definitely the way to go. Here is a short list of high GI foods. Take a look at this list and you will get a better idea as to why they feature high on the GI ranking.

- Candy and other sugary desserts are high on sugars
- White bread and foods made from white flour is highly processed
- Pasta is highly processed
- Sugary fruits like pineapple and watermelon are high on sugar

Eating a low GI diet would mean you eliminate food high in sugar, as well as unhealthy processed food and white-flour products. Instead, focus on filling your plate with lean protein, whole grains, fibrous vegetables, and some low GI fruits like berries and citrus fruits.

Glycemicindex.com will provide you with a comprehensive list of the GI values of various foods. You can enter any food you want and find out its GI value. A value of 55 or over is considered high GI. For example, white bread has a GI of 71. Ideally, you should aim to keep the value of the foods you're eating significantly below 55. Raw carrots have a GI of 35 and are considered to have a low GI.

Most of the food types listed on the low end of the glycemic index are food types that are high on fiber and low in fat. They are the right types of food to keep your heart healthy and your cholesterol low. Eating such foods will have a positive impact on your heart and your cholesterol levels, and may increase your life span with many healthy years.

If you have a family history of heart attack or stroke, you should make it a priority to know how you can take care of your heart and your health.

What you need to know about cholesterol

Cholesterol is a fat-like compound which is made in your liver and then moved through your blood. It can also be taken into your body from some food sources like meat, poultry and full-fat dairy products. You do require some cholesterol but not too much. Your liver manufactures excess cholesterol when you consume food that is high in saturated fats and trans fats.

It is often seen as a bad guy. An oversupply of this bad substance sloshing around your insides may prove to be a huge risk to your heart's health. Why, you ask, does your body manufacture something so bad for you?

It's because cholesterol also helps with some very important tasks, without which your body could suffer.

Helps to re-form cell walls

Helps your body to produce vitamin D

Helps in the creation of some steroid hormones

So why is cholesterol a problem?

When there is excessive amount of cholesterol, plaque is built up in the arteries. This makes it difficult for your blood to circulate freely and to reach your heart. That's when you get a sharp pain in your chest, which is called angina. When a plaque breaks open, it forms blood clots. You can get a heart attack when the blood supply through the artery that feeds the heart is completely blocked. If a clot clogs the blood supply to your brain, you get a stroke.

Cholesterol is oil-based. It cannot mix with the water-based blood. It needs to be transported around the body through your blood. Two types of lipoproteins facilitate this movement of cholesterol. Low-density lipoprotein or LDL carries the 'bad' cholesterol whereas high-density lipoprotein, HDL carries the 'good' cholesterol.

Even though the good and the bad cholesterol are similar in their makeup, they affect your body in different ways. It's essential to have an awareness of the levels of cholesterol in your blood. This will allow you and your doctor to figure out the best strategy to lower your risk.

Saturated fats and trans fats raise LDL levels in your blood. A surplus of LDL can be deposited on the walls of coronary arteries and lead to heart attacks. On the other hand, HDL carries cholesterol from the blood back to the liver, which processes it for elimination.

Cholesterol is not just a number. It is a ratio of the good to the bad cholesterol. When there is an increase in the amount of HDL, it carries away a lot of the bad LDL. Eating food containing trans fats not only raises the LDL but also lowers HDL. 5:1 is the commonly accepted ratio. So, for each measure of one particle of bad cholesterol, you should have at least five particles of good cholesterol in your blood.

Follow a low GI Diet for a higher level of HDL-cholesterol.

The first step that you should take to improve your cholesterol levels should be making healthy eating choices and adding 30 minutes of exercise to your day.

Increasing the HDL levels in your system actually helps lower your overall cholesterol levels. It helps to keep your arteries clear and your heart running smoothly.

What may come as a surprise to you is that the main supplier of this cholesterol to your body is the food you eat.

You are hurting yourself needlessly.

By eating food that is high in trans fats and hydrogenated fats, you are jeopardizing your own health. The GI diet will allow you to choose food that will help to lower your cholesterol, which in turn will reduce the chances of developing other health issues. The low GI food that you eat helps your body continue the business of running smoothly and keeps your heart healthy.

CHAPTER 8

The GI way to fuel your workout

The best way to boost your workout is to properly fuel your body. Your body requires specific nutrients before and after you finish your exercise routine. An optimal situation would be to keep your blood sugar level even throughout the day. This is possible if you divide your daily nutrition into smaller meals, eating a meal every two to three hours. A good understanding of the GI is key, as well.

What you eat before your workout will be useful to your body only once it has been digested and absorbed. You therefore need to time your meal or snack in such a way that the fuel is available during your workout. The amount of time needed for the food to get digested would also depend on the type and the quantity of food that is consumed.

Most foods high in fat, protein and fiber take longer to digest than other foods. Undigested food in your stomach can cause discomfort during a workout. Bigger meals take longer to digest than smaller quantities, for obvious reasons.

It has been observed that your stomach can handle food better during lower intensity activities or sports like cycling where your body gets external support, rather than in activities such as jogging or a gym workout in which your belly gets jostled a lot. It's safe to eat about 3-4 hours before your workout or enjoy a light snack about an hour or two before you begin your exercise routine.

Every individual has different needs, so play around and experiment with timing and quantities. Get to know what suits you best. See the effects on your performance and compare your exercise metabolism when you consume low or high GI food before your workout.

The GI rank of food is determined by several factors.

- The amount and type of fiber it contains. Soluble fibers have a low rating because they delay the digestion process.
- The fat and protein content in a food item also slows down the rate of digestion and has a low GI.

- GI ratings are also affected by the type of sugars the food contains. For example, maltose, a type of glucose, breaks down more rapidly when compared to fructose.
- The method of food preparation also affects the GI, for example French fries (GI of 107) take a longer time to digest when compared to baked potato (GI of 85) because they contains fats.

If you regularly exercise, it will prove advantageous to you if pay attention to a good balance of carbohydrates, including what you eat and when.

High GI Foods and your workout

When you eat food that has high GI, carbohydrates are digested faster. They cause a greater increase in blood sugar and insulin. If you want your workout to be effective, you would want to avoid high insulin levels, because insulin suppresses the utilization of fat and promotes fat storage. High GI foods include most processed cereals, potato, white bread, products made of white flour, soda, white rice, etc.

Low GI Foods and your workout

The digestion of low to moderate GI foods takes place slower. This produces a gradual rise in blood sugar. Besides the high energy levels it produces, the slow supply of blood sugar regulates the production of insulin and glucagon, two hormones which help in muscle growth and fat loss.

- Eating low GI foods reduces low blood sugar at the beginning of your workout.
- Fat oxidation increases, thereby helping to reduce dependence on carbs as fuel.
- Low GI foods provide a steady and gradual supply of blood sugar to ensure peak energy and performance.

Low GI foods include fruits like berries, pears and apples, milk, oat bran, wheat noodles, beans and legumes, broccoli, peppers, mushrooms, tomatoes etc.

Prepare for your workout.

Your body burns off stored energy very quickly during an intense workout and converts the carbohydrates into energy. Long distance runners depend on carb-loading before a marathon so they have quick acting carbohydrates accessible to fuel them through the entire run. When you don't plan and prepare, your body will burn the nutrients that are required to build muscle.

When you load up on protein and carbohydrates, make sure you increase your water consumption. Remember, water is needed for the body to store glycogen, and you should be increasing your water consumption anyway before any form of exercise or work out.

Remember to have a snack or a small meal that includes low to medium GI food and protein about an hour before you begin your workout. Some delicious choices are sweet potato casserole, warm milk or some oatmeal with nuts. It is important to give your body time to digest it and convert it into ready-to-use energy.

About half an hour before you start exercising, get a boost of immediate energy with a protein shake that has high GI fruit juices blended with whole fruit and dried figs.

After your workout

After you complete your workout, it is extremely important to refuel. You need to provide your body the required nutrients to help it recover from the workout. This post-workout nutrition should include carbohydrates and proteins. It should also be around 20% of your total caloric intake for the day.

This is the perfect time to enjoy a refreshing drink containing high GI ingredients, with both proteins and carbohydrates to increase the production of insulin. Since liquids metabolize rapidly, you can expect optimal results. A peanut butter and banana sandwich and a rolled oats smoothie with flax seeds within an hour of your workout will help you recoup faster and also build and repair muscle tissue.

At the end of the day

Your body is subjected to more stress and more spent calories on the days you work out. It is essential to make sure that your energy reserves are not depleted overnight and that your blood sugar remains level. A low GI meal with high quality protein is recommended, such as oven roasted turkey breast with a bulgur wheat salad.

The right approach to a healthy diet all day long is to maintain a balance between low GI carbohydrates and proteins. This creates a stable blood sugar level as well as a slow release of nutrients. Eating a wide variety of low GI foods gives you the best nutritional value. On the days that you work out, include a good selection of high GI foods and proteins to your diet with proper hydration.

CHAPTER 9

Following a Glycemic Index Diet is easy

The GI Diet is not hard to follow because it really isn't a diet plan. Diet plans come with so many strict rules that need to be followed; however this isn't the case with the GI Diet. The GI Diet sets down guidelines that you can follow in order to eat healthy. It is a way of life that will come to you naturally after a while. You know exactly what to eat in order to stay satiated for longer periods of time and to nourish your body in the best way.

You don't need to log every bite that you have taken; you don't need to Google each time you want to eat something new. You no longer need to be a slave to your weight loss mobile phone apps!

All you need to do is to familiarize yourself with Low GI foods and follow some general practices, you will find yourself losing weight, controlling your diabetes if you have it and benefitting from your workout routine—effortlessly.

I am not on a diet.

Accept this idea, and you'll do well. Never tell anyone that you are on a diet. You are not.

Use the GI ratings for common foods to guide you in making the best dietary choices for your day-to-day food planning. Be aware of the food types that are high on the GI list. Make a conscious effort to avoid or reduce your intake of these foods. Breakfast cereal, bagels, grape juice and pineapples are on the high list and cause an unacceptable glycemic impact you would want to avoid. Yes, they do seem like healthy food choices, so do you still need to banish these foods from your diet?

Do you need to eliminate all high GI foods?

Not as a rule. When you pair these with low GI foods, their rate of absorption in your blood stream is slow, and your hunger levels are regulated as well. For instance, when you have your breakfast cereal with milk, berries and nuts, the overall high GI effect of the cereal is reduced. Similarly, if you are yearning for a slice of cake, go ahead, and get yourself a slice of cake that has plenty of fruits and nuts and no icing.

Following a GI Diet can be exciting and fun. Spend some time looking up new GI diet recipes, and try out ones that interest you. Planning your weekly menus can be an enjoyable experience as well. When you know what you plan to eat, you could prepare a shopping list of all the ingredients you require and stock up on plenty of fresh seasonal vegetables and fruits.

Be adventurous! Try out different types of food that have low GI, food you have never tried before. Develop new favorites. You'll be surprised to find how much you enjoy the variety of foods available to you.

You could also pick up a large variety of herbs and spices. Experiment with new flavors and add new and exciting twists to your cooking. Avoid deep frying your food in oils; choose cooking methods like boiling, baking or steaming.

Remember, portion sizes are important. Just because an ingredient has low GI, don't over eat. Larger portion size increases the work load on your system, releasing more insulin into your blood stream.

CHAPTER 10

Planning a Glycemic Index Diet meal

Now that you have almost reached the end of this ebook, I'm sure you would agree that a low GI diet is a healthy, balanced diet that can suit anyone. When you follow a GI Diet, you are able to reduce the feeling of being hungry between meals. When you have reduced your hunger pangs, you automatically reduce the feeling of being starved and avoid making unhealthy eating choices. A low GI diet also benefits people with diabetes or those who are struggling to lose weight.

When you are planning a low GI diet plan, you must try and chose recipes that are high in fiber and low on the GI ranking scale. When you think of low GI foods, think of whole grain breads, grains and cereals, low GI fruits and starchy vegetables and zero processed foods.

I have below a few suggestions on how you can plan a meal. Feel free to add in your own meals and snacks. However, it is best to stay clear of highly processed foods. It's quite easy to do that—just avoid walking through the aisle in the supermarket which contains food packaged in plastic. Instead, buy real, fresh produce. You would be doing yourself and the environment a great favor. Also, try to avoid sodas, fruit juices and sweets as much as you can.

Start your day with a wholesome Low GI breakfast.

Breakfasts for most of us bring to mind the sounds of a toaster popping, the gurgle of juice being poured into a glass, crunching muesli, or the hum of low conversations as people queue up for their cream cheese bagels. Traditionally, popular breakfast foods are carbohydrate-based.

Popular high GI breakfast foods like white bread, bagels, cereals, as well as juices, spike your blood sugar and leave you feeling hungry. Starting the day out with low GI options helps stabilize your blood sugar all morning and keeps you feeling fuller until lunch time.

Healthy, low GI breakfast ideas

1 slice of whole grain bread or 50 gm of traditional porridge made from old-fashioned oats or bran flakes cereal

High protein food such as eggs and cheese

One small bowl of skimmed milk or yogurt

Choose peanut butter instead of butter

Whole fruits like berries or citrus fruits like oranges

Decaffeinated coffee, tea and water

Low GI breakfast recipes

One-pan egg delight

Ingredients:

1 tbsp olive oil

2 medium sized zucchinis, chopped into medium sized cubes

5-6 cherry tomatoes, halved

2 garlic cloves, crushed

2 eggs

basil leaves, to serve

Method:

1. Heat olive oil slightly in a frying pan and add the zucchini.
2. Stir fry for 5 minutes.
3. When it starts to soften, add the tomatoes and garlic then cook for a few minutes more. Add in some salt and pepper.
4. Make some space within this mix and break in the eggs. Cover and cook for 2-3 minutes until the eggs are done.
5. Scatter some basil leaves and serve with whole grain bread, an orange and a cup of decaffeinated coffee or tea.

Fruity Nutty porridge

Ingredients:

50g steel cut oats, soaked overnight
Mixed dry fruits including raisins, dates, walnuts, figs and almonds

1 ½ cups (350ml) skimmed milk or water

Method:

1. Put the oats in a saucepan; pour in the milk or water.
2. Bring to boil and simmer for 4-5 minutes, stirring from time to time. Remove from heat.
3. Add the dry fruits and leave to stand for 2 minutes before eating.

Protein up your Lunch.

Protein foods have zero carbs, so they are zero on the GI scale. Fill your plate with protein-rich foods like tuna, turkey, chicken, cheese or eggs. If you are vegan or vegetarian, some low GI lunch options include tofu and legumes such as black beans, kidney beans, lentils, or chickpeas. Always choose whole grain versions of food like bread, pasta and rice.

Watch out for sneaky, hidden sources of high GI products, which could take the form of mayonnaise within your multi-grain sandwiches or your salads drenched in salad dressings and condiments that have added sugar and sweeteners.

Protein rich low GI lunch ideas

Chili with beans served with organic brown rice pilaf and some fruit for dessert.

Spring salad (no dressings) with oil and vinegar on the side.

Home-made soups containing lentils served with a whole grain roll.

Whole meal bread sandwich with hummus or turkey fillings served with a cold chicken salad.

Thick cauliflower soup with a small bowl of couscous flavored with lemon and herbs.

Low GI lunch recipes

Chicken & beans medley

Ingredients:

1 tbsp olive oil

2 skinless chicken thighs

1 onion, chopped

2 garlic cloves, chopped

1/2 tsp dried thyme

1 cup (250ml) white wine

1 lb fava beans in their pods, shelled

Parsley leaves, to garnish

Method:

1. Heat olive oil in a frying pan. Add the chicken, and cook till brown.
2. Now add the onion, garlic and thyme, and fry for 2 minutes. Pour in the wine and 2 cups of water and season with salt and pepper to taste. Allow to boil, and simmer for 20 minutes, covering for the first 10 minutes. Cook till the chicken is tender.
3. Stir the fava beans in and continue to cook, stirring occasionally, until tender, about 3 minutes. Scatter roughly chopped parsley, and serve with long grain basmati rice.

Vegetable Casserole

Ingredients:

1 can of cream of mushroom soup

1 cup chopped broccoli

1 cup cauliflower florets

1 cup mushrooms, sliced

1 cup of mixed vegetables like peas, yellow and red peppers

6 ounce pack of soy cheese

Method:

1. Mix all the vegetables listed above with the mushroom soup.
2. Pour half of the mixture on the bottom of a baking pan.
3. Spread the soy cheese as the second layer. Pour the rest of the vegetable mixture on top.
4. Preheat oven to 340 F (170 C) and bake casserole for 30 minutes.
5. Enjoy after letting it rest for 10 minutes.

Mind the starches at your dinner table.

It's best to stay away from starchy food at dinner. If you like to eat rice, potatoes or pasta, eat it as the side dish rather than as the main dish. Better choices would include brown rice, boiled potatoes or whole wheat pasta, because these items are less processed. When you eat these food items, your body has to work extra hard and longer in order to break it down, so energy will be released much slower.

Feel free to eat lean cuts of meat or fish since these have a high protein content, and therefore, are carb free. Pile your plate high with salads, and non-starchy vegetables that are low to medium GI.

Think outside the box.

If you have had a very busy day, and are tired to the bone, you really don't have to spend hours preparing a traditional dinner recipe. You may want to avoid reach for the take-out menu to order a greasy meal that contains mystery ingredients. Instead, make wholesome, simple fare like an omelet with French toast using 100% whole wheat bread. A nutritious sweet potato hash with vegetables and shredded turkey breast is very easy to make and has low GI as well. Chop up portions of all the low GI veggies in your refrigerator and prepare a warming, nutritious, low GI bowl of soup that you could enjoy with a dinner roll or salad. Finish your dinner with some fruit and cheese, instead of sugary desserts that would immediately raise your blood sugar, and spoil your chances of a deep, undisturbed sleep later that night.

Low GI dinner recipes

Baked Salmon with crunchy nut topping

Ingredients:

16 ounces (500 gms) salmon fillet
½ cup breadcrumbs
Chopped parsley
2 ounces (50 gms) almonds, chopped
2 ounces (50 gms) walnuts, chopped

1 tablespoon fresh lemon juice
1 avocado, sliced
2 tbsp olive oil
Salt and pepper to taste

Method

Preheat oven to 350 F (175 C) and place fish on baking tray. Mix breadcrumbs, parsley, almonds, walnuts and lemon juice. Add salt and pepper to taste. Spread over each piece of fish and drizzle some olive oil. Bake for 5 minutes, not allowing the fish to overcook. Toss the avocado with oil and lemon juice and serve with fish.

Sweet potato and black bean stew

Ingredients:

2 red onions, diced

2 tbsp olive oil

1 ½ ounces (50 g) ginger, pounded

1 vegetable stock cube, crumbled

1 lb (500 gms) sweet potatoes, peeled and chopped into cubes

Small bunch cilantro, leaves only

5 tomatoes, pureed

2 tbsp vinegar

½ lb (200 gms) black beans, boiled

Green peppers, to taste

Method:

1. Heat olive oil in a frying pan and sauté the diced onion.
2. Add in the pounded ginger, pureed tomatoes and the crumbled vegetable stock cube.
3. Add 2 cups (500 ml) water and bring to a simmer.
4. Add the sweet potatoes and cook till soft.
5. Now add the boiled black beans and the peppers. Scatter chopped cilantro leaves and serve.

CHAPTER 11

Foods and Their Glycemic Index

Below you will find the glycemic index rating for 150 various foods.
Low GI = 55 or less
Medium GI = 56 - 69
High GI = 70 or more

Breakfast Cereal Glycemic Index

Low GI

All-bran (UK/Aus) 30

All-bran (US) 50

Oat bran 50

Rolled Oats 51

Special K (UK/Aus) 54

Natural Muesli 40

Porridge 58

Medium GI

Bran Buds 58

Mini Wheats 58

Nutrigrain 66

Shredded Wheat 67

Porridge Oats 63

Special K (US) 69

High GI

Cornflakes 80

Sultana Bran 73

Bran flakes 74

Coco Pops 77

Puffed Wheat 80

Oats in Honey Bake 77

Team 82

Total 76

Cheerios 74

Rice Krispies 82

Weetabix 74

Bread

Low GI
Soya and Linseed   36
Wholegrain Pumpernickel   46
Heavy Mixed Grain   45
Whole Wheat   49

Sourdough Rye   48
Sourdough Wheat   54

Medium GI
Croissant   67
Hamburger bun   61

Pita, white   57
Whole meal Rye   62

High GI
White   71
Bagel   72

French Baguette   95

Staples

Low GI
Wheat Pasta Shapes   54
New Potatoes   54
Meat Ravioli   39
Spaghetti   32
Tortellini (Cheese)   50
Egg Fettuccini   32
Brown Rice   50

Buckwheat   51
White long grain rice   50
Pearled Barley   22
Yam   35
Sweet Potatoes   48
Instant Noodles   47
Wheat tortilla   30

Medium GI
Basmati Rice   58
Couscous   61
Cornmeal   68
Taco Shells   68
Gnocchi   68

Canned Potatoes   61
Chinese (Rice) Vermicelli   58
Baked Potatoes   60
Wild Rice   57

High GI
Instant White Rice   87
Glutinous Rice   86
Short Grain White Rice   83
Tapioca   70

Fresh Mashed Potatoes   73
French Fries   75
Instant Mashed Potatoes   80

Snacks & Sweet Foods

Low GI

Slim-Fast meal replacement 27
Snickers Bar (high fat) 41
Nut & Seed Muesli Bar 49
Sponge Cake 46
Nutella 33
Milk Chocolate 42
Hummus 6

Peanuts 13
Walnuts 15
Cashew Nuts 25
Nuts and Raisins 21
Jam 51
Corn Chips 42
Oatmeal Crackers 55

Medium GI

Ryvita 63
Digestives 59

Blueberry muffin 59
Honey 58

High GI

Pretzels 83
Water Crackers 78
Rice cakes 87
Puffed Crisp bread 81

Donuts 76
Scones 92
Maple flavored syrup 68

Vegetables

Low GI

Frozen Green Peas 39
Frozen Sweet Corn 47
Raw Carrots 16
Boiled Carrots 41
Eggplant/Aubergine 15
Broccoli 10
Cauliflower 15
Cabbage 10

Mushrooms 10
Tomatoes 15
Chiles 10
Lettuce 10
Green Beans 15
Red Peppers 10
Onions 10

Medium GI

Beetroot 64

High GI

Pumpkin 75

Parsnips 97

Fruits

Low GI

Cherries 22

Plums 24

Grapefruit 25

Peaches 28

Peach, canned in natural juice 30

Apples 34

Pears 41

Dried Apricots 32

Grapes 43

Coconut 45

Coconut Milk 41

Kiwi Fruit 47

Oranges 40

Strawberries 40

Prunes 29

Medium GI

Mango 60

Sultanas 56

Bananas 58

Raisins 64

Papaya 60

Figs 61

Pineapple 66

High GI

Watermelon 80

Dates 103

Legumes (Beans)

Low GI

Kidney Beans (canned) 52

Butter Beans 36

Chick Peas 42

Haricot/Navy Beans 31

Lentils, Red 21

Lentils, Green 30

Pinto Beans 45

Black-eyed Beans 50

Yellow Split Peas 32

Medium GI

Beans in Tomato Sauce 56

Dairy

Low GI

Whole milk 31

Skimmed milk 32

Chocolate milk 42

Sweetened yogurt 33

Artificially Sweetened Yogurt 23

Custard 35

Soy Milk 44

Medium GI
Ice Cream   62

Chart courtesy of the University of Sydney.

Conclusion

Thank you again for downloading this book!

I hope this book was able to help you to understand how you can monitor the types of food you eat based on the glycemic index (GI) and improve your health to assist your body to function more naturally.

The next step is to follow the guidelines recommended in this book. You will soon come to realize that it comes effortlessly once you become familiar with it. The GI diet does not prohibit you from eating any food that you like or count calories; it only recommends that you regulate your meals and make the best choice you can in most situations. Your body deserves it.

Finally, if you enjoyed this book, then I'd like to ask you for a favor, would you be kind enough to leave a review for this book on Amazon? It'd be greatly appreciated!

Be sure to check out our website at www.thetotalevolution.com for more information.

Thank you!

Our Other Books

Below you'll find some of our other books that are popular on Amazon.com and the international sites.

Master Cleanse: How To Do A Natural Detox The Right Way And Lose Weight Fast

Mayo Clinic Diet: A Proven Diet Plan For Lifelong Weight Loss

Dukan Diet: A High Protein Diet Plan To Lose Weight And Keep It Off For Life

Clean Eating Diet: A 10 Day Diet Plan To Eat Clean, Lose Weight And Supercharge Your Body

Wheat Belly: The Anti-Diet - A Guide To Gluten Free Eating And A Slimmer Belly

IIFYM: Flexible Dieting - Sculpt The Perfect Body While Eating The Foods You Love

Mediterranean Diet: 101 Ultimate Mediterranean Diet Recipes To Fast Track Your Weight Loss & Help Prevent Disease

Acid Reflux Diet: A Beginner's Guide To Natural Cures And Recipes For Acid Reflux, GERD And Heartburn

Hypothyroidism Diet: Natural Remedies & Foods To Boost Your Energy & Jump Start Your Weight Loss

It Starts With Food: A 30 Day Diet Plan To Reset Your Body, Lose Weight And Become A Healthier You

CPSIA information can be obtained
at www.ICGtesting.com
Printed in the USA
LVHW111811060120
642663LV00001BA/349/P

9 781519 214973